COMPETENCY BASED LOGBOOK

for

ANM

(कम्पीटेन्सी बेस्ड लॉगबुक फॉर एएनएम)

(*As per the revised INC syllabus*)
(*Hindi and English*)

COMPETENCY BASED LOGBOOK

for

ANM

(कम्पीटेन्सी बेस्ड लॉगबुक फॉर एएनएम)

(*As per the revised INC syllabus*)
(*Hindi and English*)

NAME OF THE CANDIDATE : --

EXAMINATION ROLL NUMBER : --

NAME OF THE INSTITUTE : --

ACADEMIC YEAR : ---------------------- **To** --------------------

COMPETENCY BASED LOGBOOK

for

ANM

(कम्पीटेन्सी बेस्ड लॉगबुक फॉर एएनएम)

(*As per the revised INC syllabus*)
(*Hindi and English*)

Vijaya Santhi Murugesan MSc (N) (Community Health)
Principal
Combined (P.G) Institute of Medical Sciences & Research
Haridwar Road, Dehradun
Uttarakhand, India

JAYPEE

JAYPEE BROTHERS MEDICAL PUBLISHERS

The Health Sciences Publisher

New Delhi | London

Jaypee Brothers Medical Publishers (P) Ltd

Headquarters
Jaypee Brothers Medical Publishers (P) Ltd
23/23-B, Ansari Road, Daryaganj
New Delhi 110 002, India
Phone: +91-11-23272143, +91-11-23272703
+91-11-23282021, +91-11-23245672
E-mail: jaypee@jaypeebrothers.com

Corporate Office
Jaypee Brothers Medical Publishers (P) Ltd.
4838/24, Ansari Road, Daryaganj
New Delhi 110 002, India
Phone: +91-11-43574357
Fax: +91-11-43574314
E-mail: jaypee@jaypeebrothers.com

Overseas Office
J P Medical Ltd
83 Victoria Street, London
SW1H 0HW (UK)
Phone: +44 20 3170 8910
E-mail: info@jpmedpub.com

EU GPSR Authorised Representative
Logos Europe, 9 rue Nicolas Poussin
17000, La Rochelle, France
Phone: +33 (0) 6 67 93 73 78
E-mail: Contact@logoseurope.eu

Website: www.jaypeebrothers.com
Website: www.jaypeedigital.com

Competency Based Logbook for ANM (कम्पीटेन्सी बेस्ड लॉगबुक फॉर एएनएम)

First Edition: 2014

Reprint : **2025**

ISBN : 978-93-5152-208-9

Printed in India at Sterling Graphics Pvt. Ltd.

Preface

"Knock the door, it will be opened;

Ask, it will be given;

Search, you will find"

"Be thirsty to fulfil your thirstiness (learning)"

It gives me immense pleasure to guide the clinical supervisor, community field supervisor and the ANM students through this Logbook, to meet all the clinical competency.

The first edition of the Logbook is developed by myself to maintain uniformity and unanimity among the nursing institution throughout our whole nation.

Community Health Nurses (CHNs) are the basic unit of the health and Family Welfare Programmes, at all levels of Health Care Delivery System. In our country, ANMs are holding the role and responsibilities of the community health nurse. So it is necessary that, the ANMs, should have adequate knowledge and competencies to provide comprehensive, promotive and preventive health services to the individual, family and community in both rural and urban areas without any discrimination and negligence.

I assure that, this Logbook will provide the maximum support to fulfil the requirements of ANM course as per the revised Indian Nursing Council Syllabus.

Vijaya Santhi Murugesan

Acknowledgements

- It is a great blessing from GOD that he has given me good parents and chairman Dr GS Jadaun, MD (Patho), who motivated and supported me very well in preparing this Logbook.
- I acknowledge, my thankfulness to Dr Tarun Chandana MD, Director (Academic). And I am sincerely thankful to Dr Bahuguna MBBS, DCP, Ex CMO for his valuable support in translation and correction of the Logbook in Hindi.
- And also I express my heartfelt thanks to Ms Daljeet Kaur Sudan MSc(N) for her great help in translation of the Logbook in Hindi.
- I am very much proud and thankful to my parents Mr Murugesan, and Mrs Rajaveni for their constant and consistent support to bring me in this profession. And I am immensely grateful to My Brother Dr Vijay Srinivasan, MSc, MPhil, PhD, for his moral support.
- Here I want to express my beloved thanks to my husband Mr Joseph Peter, MA, (English and Sociology) and my son Master. Karlfred Niranjan and my daughter Nirai Mathi for their cooperations in preparing this Logbook.
- I extend my sincere thanks to the editorial board of M/s Jaypee Brothers Medical Publishers (P) Ltd New Delhi, Mr Bhupesh Arora (General Manager -Publishing), Mrs Preeti Parashar (Author Coordinator) and Mr Rishi Sourabh Sharma for completing this work and publishing this logbook successfully.

Contents

(विषय-सूची)

INC PRESCRIBED PRACTICAL HOURS

S. No	SUBJECTS	CLASSROOM DEMONSTRATIONS (Hours)	CLINICAL EXPERIENCE (Hours)		
			HOSPTIAL	COMMUINITY	TOTAL
FIRST YEAR					
I	**Community Health Nursing**	50	10	100	110
II	**Health Promotion**	75	20	180	200
A	Nutrition	30			
B	Human Body and Hygiene	20			
C	Environmental Sanitation	15			
D	Mental Health	10			
III	**Primary Health Care Nursing-I**	150	90	300	390
A	Infection and Immunization	20			
B	Communicable Disease	25			
C	Community Health Problems	50			
D	Primary Medical Care	20			
E	First Aid and Referral	35			
IV	**Child Health Nursing**	110	80	100	180
	TOTAL HOURS	385	200	680	880
SECOND YEAR					
V	**Midwifery**	160	220	160	380
VI	**Health Center Management**	40		60	60
	TOTAL HOURS	200	220	220	440
INTERNSHIP PEROID					
I	**Midwifery**		240	240	480
	Antenatal Ward		40		
	Intranatal/Lobor Room		120		
	Postnatal Ward		40		
	Neonatal Ward		40		
II	**Child Health Nursing**		80	160	240
III	**Community Health and Health Center Management**			160	160
	TOTAL HOURS		320	560	380

COMPETENCIES

S. No	Competencies (कार्यनिर्वाह क्षमताएँ)	Number of Requirement
I	**COMMUNITY HEALTH NURSING** (सामुदायिक स्वास्थ्य परिचर्या)	
1	Survey (सर्वेक्षण)	3
2	Mapping (मानचित्र बनाना)	3
3	Prepare Health Organization Chart (स्वास्थ्य संगठन चार्ट बनाना)	2
4	Home Visit (Family Health Assessment) होम विज़िट (पारिवारिक स्वास्थ्य का आंकलन)	5
5	Community Need Assessment (सामुदायिक आवश्यकताओं का आंकलन)	1
6	Bag Technique (बैग तकनीक)	10
7	Oral Rehydration Therapy (ORT) (मौखिक पुर्नजलीकरण थेरेपी)	1
8	Assess Personal Hygiene of School Children (स्कूली बच्चों की व्यक्तिगत स्वच्छता का आंकलन)	5
9	Preparation of IEC Material (आई0ई0सी0 सामिग्री की तैयारी)	7
10	Conduct BCC Session (Role Play/folk Method) बी0सी0सी0सत्र का संचालन (रोल प्ले/फोल्क मेथड)	1
11	Prepare Health Education Plan (स्वास्थ्य शिक्षा योजना बनाना)	1
12	Health Education (स्वास्थ्य शिक्षा)	3
13	Counselling (समाधान)	2
14	Participate in Health and Family Welfare Programme (स्वास्थ्य एवं परिवार कल्याण कार्यक्रम मे भाग लेना)	1
15	Field Visit (ग्रामीण क्षैत्र का दौरा)	7
16	Group Work (सामूहिक कार्य)	3
II	**HEALTH PROMOTION** (स्वास्थ्य का विकास)	
A	**NUTRITION** (पोषण)	
1	Nutritional Assessment (पोषण का आंकलन)	2

S. No	Competencies (कार्यनिर्वाह क्षमताएँ)	Number of Requirement
2	Diet Planning (भोजन की योजना)	2
3	Cooking Special Diet (विशेष भोजन पकाना)	1
4	Nutrition Education to a Group (एक समूह को पोषण शिक्षा)	1
5	Counselling on Nutrition (पोषण पर काउन्सिलिंग)	3
6	Exhibition on Balanced Diet (Using Raw Food Items) संतुलित आहार पर प्रदर्शनी (कच्चे खाद्य पदार्थो का प्रयोग)	1
7	Observational Visit (ओबजर्वेशनल विजिट)	2
B	**HUMAN BODY & HYGIENE** (मानव शरीर एवं स्वच्छता)	
8	Preparation of Anatomy Practical Book (एनाटमी की प्रैक्टिकल बुक बनाना)	1
9	Care of Various Parts of Sick (रोगी के विभिन्न अंगो की देखभाल)	5
10	Health Education on Menstrual Hygiene (मासिक चक्र के समय स्वच्छता पर स्वास्थ्य शिक्षा)	1
11	Counselling the Adolescence on Physiological Changes, Fulfillment of Basic Needs, Body Hygiene, and Healthy Life Styles (किशोरो को शारीरिक बदलाव, मूल आवश्यकताओं की भरपाई, शारीरिक स्वच्छता, एवं स्वास्थ्यप्रद जीवनशैली पर काउन्सिलिंग)	1
C	**ENVIRONMENTAL SANITATION** (वातावरण की स्वच्छता)	
12	Village Mapping (Water Source, Drains, Ponds & Contaminated Areas) गाँव का मानचित्र (जल स्रोत, नालिया तालाब एवं गन्दे क्षेत्र)	1
13	Demonstrate Purification of Water (जल का शुद्धिकरण सिखाना)	2
14	Guide or Plan Construction on Small Scale Soak Pit at School or Health Center (स्कूल या स्वास्थ्य केन्द्र पर छोटे स्केल का सोकपिट बनाने पर मार्गदर्शन या योजना बनाना)	1
15	Health Education on use of Sanitary Latrine (सैनिट्री लैट्रिन के प्रयोग हेतु स्वास्थ्य शिक्षा)	1
16	Field Visit (फील्ड विजिट)	2
D	**MENTAL HEALTH** (मानसिक स्वास्थ्य)	
17	Assessment of Mental Health Status of an Individual (व्यक्ति के मानसिक स्वास्थ्य स्तर का आंकलन)	2

S. No	Competencies (कार्यनिर्वाह क्षमताएँ)	Number of Requirement
18	Care of Mentally Challenged Patient (मानसिक रोगी की देखभाल)	1
19	Counselling of Maladjusted Individual in Community (समुदाय मे मालएडजस्टेड व्यक्ति की काउन्सिलिंग)	1
20	Care Plan for an Elderly Person at Home (एक वृद्धव्यक्ति की घर पर देखभाल की योजना)	1
21	Observational Visit (ओबजर्वेशनल विजिट)	2
III	**PRIMARY HEALTH CARE-I** (प्राथमिक स्वास्थ्य देखभाल भाग-I)	
A	**INFECTION AND IMMUNIZATION** (संक्रमण एवं टीकाकरण)	
1	Sterilisation of Syringes and Needles (Using Pressure Cooker/Small Autoclave) सिरिंज एवं सुईयों का विसंक्रमण (प्रेशर कुकर/छोटे ओटोक्लेव के प्रयोग से)	1
2	Vaccination Technique (टीकाकरण तकनीक)	1
3	Assisting or Participating in Cold Chain System (शीतश्रृँखला प्रणाली में भागेदारी या सहायता)	5
4	Participating in Immunization Camp (टीकाकरण कैम्प मे भाग लेना)	1
5	Maintenance of Immunization Record (टीकाकरण रिकार्ड का रखरखाव)	1
6	Preparation of Posture or Chart on Immunization Schedule (टीकाकरण सारिणी पर पोस्टर या चार्ट बनाना)	1
7	Preparation of Malarial Slides (मलेरियल स्लाईडस बनाना)	1
8	Collection of Specimen (स्पेसीमेन इक्ठ्ठा करना)	4
9	Biomedical Waste Management (जैव चिकित्सा अपशिष्ट का प्रबंधन)	1
B	**COMMUNICABLE DISEASE** (संक्रमण रोग)	
10	Calculation of Morbidity and Mortality Rate (रूग्णता एवं मृत्यु दर की गणना)	1
11	Preparation of Surveillance Report (सर्वेलेन्स रिपोर्ट बनाना)	1
12	Standard Safety Measures in Nursing Practice (नर्सिंग प्रैक्टिस में स्टैन्डर्ड सेफ्टी मेज़र्स)	1
13	Prepare Chart on Standard Safety Measures (स्टैन्डर्ड सेफ्टी मेज़र्स का चार्ट बनाना)	1

S. No	Competencies (कार्यनिर्वाह क्षमताएँ)	Number of Requirement
14	Care of Communicable Disease (Child/Adult) (संक्रामक रोग की देखभाल बच्चे/वयस्क)	2
15	Participate in Control of Epidemic and its Relief Work in the Community (समुदाय मे महामारी के बचाव कार्य तथा नियंत्रण में भाग लेना)	1
16	Conduct Health Education on Communicable Disease (संक्रामक रोग पर स्वास्थ्य शिक्षा का संचालन)	1
17	Observational Visit (ओबजर्वेशनल विज़िट)	2
C	**COMMUNITY HEALTH PROBLEMS** (सामुदायिक स्वास्थ्य कठिनाईयाँ)	
18	Vital Signs and BP (जैविक चिन्ह एवं बी0पी0)	1
19	Urine Testing (मूत्र जाँच)	2
20	Steam Inhalation (स्टीम इन्हेलेशन)	1
21	Oxygen Inhalation (ऑक्सीजन इन्हेलेशन)	1
22	Instillation of Nasal drops (नेजल ड्राप्स् डालना)	1
23	Instillation of Eye drops (नेत्र ड्राप्स् डालना)	1
24	Local Hot Application (लोकल हॉट एप्लीकेशन)	1
25	Local Cold Application (लोकल कोल्ड एप्लीकेशन)	1
26	Urinary Catheterisation (यूरीनरी केथेटेराइजेशन)	1
27	Plain Water Enema (प्लेन वॉटर एनीमा)	1
28	Case Study on Patient (रोगियो पर केस अध्ययन)	5
D	**PRIMARY MEDICAL CARE** (प्राथमिक चिकित्सा से देखभाल)	
29	Calculation of Drug Dose & Conversion (ड्रग डोज़ का अनुमान एवं परिवर्तन करना)	1
30	Preparation of List of Common Drug used in Sub Centre (Dosage, Route and Action, Indication, Contraindication, Side Effect) उपकेन्द्र में उपयोग होने वाली दवाईयों की सूची बनाना (दवा की मात्रा, कहाँ से देना, प्रभाव)	1

S. No	Competencies (कार्यनिर्वाह क्षमताएँ)	Number of Requirement
31	Administration of Medicine (दवाईयों का एडमिनिस्ट्रेशन)	7
32	Preparation & Administration of IV fluids (आई0वी0 द्रव की तैयारी करना एवं देना)	3
33	Preparation of Blood Transfusion as per the Protocol (नियमों के अनुसार रक्त चढाने की तैयारी)	1
34	Drug Study (दवाईयो का अध्ययन)	3
35	Participate in AYUSH Activity (आयुष कार्यवाही मे भाग लेना)	1
E	**FIRST AID & REFERRAL** (प्राथमिक सहायता एवं संदर्भण)	
36	Care of Wound (घाव की देखभाल)	1
37	Applications (लगाने की विधि)	5
38	Insertion of Nasogastric Tube and Stomach Wash (नेसोगेसट्रिक ट्यूब डालना तथा स्टमक वॉश)	1
39	Emergency Care (आपातकालीन देखभाल)	3
40	Basic Life Support (BLS) (बेसिक लाईफ सपोर्ट बी0एल0एस0)	1
41	Transportation of Casualties (मरीजों का परिवहन)	1
IV. A	**CHILD HEALTH NURSING (HOSPITAL)** शिशु स्वास्थ्य परिचर्या (अस्पताल)	
1	Assess the Growth and Development of Children and Record on Chart (बच्चों की वृद्धि एवं विकास का आंकलन तथा चार्ट पर रिकार्ड)	10
2	Assess the Health Status of Sick Children (बीमार बच्चों के स्वास्थ्य स्तर पर आंकलन)	10
3	Care of Common Childhood Illness (as per the IMNCI Protocol) बचपन के सामान्य रोगों की देखभाल (आई0एम0एन0सी0आई0 नियमों के अनुसार)	10
4	Infection Prevention Practice (संक्रमण रोकथाम प्रैक्टिस)	3
5	Care of Child Immunization (बच्चें के टीकाकरण की देखभाल)	6
IV. B	**CHILD HEALTH NURSING (COMMUNITY)** शिशु स्वास्थ्य परिचर्या (समुदाय)	
6	Assess the Growth and Development of Children and Record on Chart (बच्चों की वृद्धि एवं विकास का आंकलन तथा चार्ट पर रिकार्ड)	10

S. No	Competencies (कार्यनिर्वाह क्षमताएँ)	Number of Requirement
7	Assess the Health Status of Sick Children (बीमार बच्चों के स्वास्थ्य स्तर का आंकलन)	10
8	Assess the Nutritional Status of the Children (बच्चों के पोषण स्तर का आंकलन)	2
9	Home Care of Common Childhood Illness (as per the IMNCI Protocol) बचपन मे होने वाले सामान्य रोगों की घर पर देखभाल (आई0एम0एन0सी0आई0 नियमों के अनुसार)	10
10	Identify and Refer the Children at Risk (रिस्क वाले बच्चों को पहचानना एवं रेफर करना)	1
11	Infection Prevention Practice (संक्रमण निरोधक प्रैक्टिस)	2
12	Health Education (स्वास्थ्य शिक्षा)	6
13	Prepare Poster (पोस्टर बनाना)	4
14	Counselling (काउन्सिलिंग)	3
15	Survey on Child Labour in the Community (समुदाय में बाल मजदूरी पर सर्वेक्षण)	1
16	Observational Visit to School (स्कूल पर ओबजर्वेशनल विजिट)	1
17	Organise or Participate in School Health Service (स्कूल स्वास्थ्य सेवाओं मे भागेदारी या संगठन)	1
18	Maintain School Health Record (स्कूल स्वास्थ्य रिकार्ड बनाना)	5
19	Case Studies (Hospital/Community) केस स्टडीज़ (अस्पताल / समुदाय)	4
V	MIDWIFERY (प्रसूति विद्या)	
A.1	CARE OF ANTENATAL MOTHERS IN HOSPITAL (अस्पताल में गर्भवती माताओं की देखभाल)	
1	Pre Conception Counselling (गर्भधारण से पूर्व काउन्सिलिंग)	2
2	Detecting Pregnancy by using Pregnancy Testing Kit (गर्भ जाँच किट के प्रयोग से गर्भ का पता लगाना)	2
3	Calculation of EDD (ई0डी0डी0 अनुमान लगाना)	2
4	Registration of Antenatal Mothers (प्रसव से पूर्व माताओं का पंजीकरण)	2
5	Hemoglobin Estimation (हीमोग्लोबिन की जाँच)	2

S. No	Competencies (कार्यनिर्वाह क्षमताएँ)	Number of Requirement
6	Urine Test (मूत्र जाँच)	2
7	Antenatal Examination प्रसव पूर्व परीक्षण	15
8	Supplementation of IFA (Iron & Folic Acid) आई0एफ0ए0 के पूरक (आयरन एवं फॉलिक एसिड)	10
9	Administration of TT Injection (टी0टी0 इंजेक्शन लगाना)	10
A.2	CARE OF ANTENATAL MOTHERS IN COMMUNITY (समुदाय में गर्भवती माताओं की देखभाल करना)	
10	Registration of Vital Events Registers (जैविक घटनाओं के रजिस्टर का पंजीकरण)	1
11	Assist in Management of Vital Events Registers (जैविक घटनाओं के रजिस्टर के प्रबंधन में सहायता)	1
12	Participate in Antenatal Clinics in the Sub Center (उपकेन्द्र पर एंटीनेटल क्लिनिक मे भाग लेना)	1
13	Antenatal Examination (प्रसवपूर्व परीक्षण)	5
14	Malaria Testing for Pregnant Mothers (गर्भवती माताओं की मलेरिया जाँच)	1
15	Counselling (काउन्सिलिंग)	7
B	INTRANATAL CARE IN HOSPITAL AND COMMUNITY (अस्पताल व समुदाय में गर्भवती माताओं की देखभाल)	
16	Maintain Midwifery Case Book (मिडवाइफरी केस बुक बनाना)	1
17	Assessment and Care of First Stage of Labour (PV Examination) (प्रसव के पहले चरण का आंकलन एवं देखभाल (पी0वी0 परीक्षण)	5
18	Plotting the Partograph (पोर्टोग्राफ भरना)	5
19	Assessment and Care of Second and Third Stage of Labour – Conducting Safe Deliveries (प्रसव के दूसरे तथा तीसरे चरण का आंकलन तथा देखभाल)	10
20	Assist in the Suturing (Episiotomies and Tears) टांके लगाने में सहायता (एपीजियोटमी एवं टीयर)	5
21	Assist in Management of Intranatal Complications (प्रसवोत्तर जटिलताओं के प्रबंधन मे सहायता)	1
C.1	CARE OF POSTNATAL MOTHERS IN HOSPITAL (अस्पताल में प्रसव के बाद माताओं की देखभाल)	
22	Provide Essential Care of the Newborn (नवजात को अतिआवश्यक देखभाल प्रदान करना)	10

S. No	Competencies (कार्यनिर्वाह क्षमताएँ)	Number of Requirement
23	Basic Resuscitation of the Newborn (नवजात का बेसिक रिससीटेशन)	5
24	Care of Postnatal Mothers (प्रसव के बाद माताओं की देखभाल)	10
25	Health Education (स्वास्थ्य शिक्षा)	6
26	Counselling (काउन्सिलिंग)	3
27	Follow Biomedical Waste Management (जैव कचरा प्रबंधन)	2
C.2	**CARE OF POSTNATAL MOTHERS IN COMMUNITY** (समुदाय में प्रसव के बाद माताओं की देखभाल)	
28	Follow-up of Postnatal Mothers (प्रसव के बाद माताओं की देखभाल)	10
29	Care of Newborn (नवजात की देखभाल)	10
30	Conduct Health Education (स्वास्थ्य शिक्षा का संचालन)	4
D.1	**IDENTIFY HIGH –RISK MOTHERS AND GIVE CARE IN HOSPITAL** (अस्पताल में अधिक जोखिम वर्ग वाली माताओं को पहचानना तथा देखभाल करना)	
31	Identify High-risk Mothers and Give Care (अधिक जोखिम वर्ग वाली माताओं को पहचानना तथा देखभाल करना)	2
32	Prepare for Caesarean Sections (सिज़ेरियन सेक्शन की तैयारी)	2
33	Observe Caesarean Section (सिज़ेरियन सेक्शन देखना)	2
34	Observe Abnormal Deliveries (असाधारण प्रसव देखना)	5
35	Prepare for MTP and Observe Procedure (एम0टी0पी0 की तैयारी तथा प्रोसीजर देखना)	2
36	Care of Women with Abortion (गर्भपात वाली महिलाओं की देखभाल)	2
37	Starting Intravenous Line (इंट्रावीनस लाईन शुरू करना)	2
38	Urinary Catheterisation in Women (महिलाओं में युरीनरी कैथेटेराइजेशन)	2
39	Preparation and Administration of Magnesium Sulphate Injection (मैग्निशियम सल्फेट इंजेक्शन तैयार करना तथा लगाना)	1

S. No	Competencies (कार्यनिर्वाह क्षमताएँ)	Number of Requirement
40	Preparation and Administration of Oxytocin Drip (आक्सीटोसिन ड्रिप तैयार करना तथा देना)	1
41	Assist/Observe Bimanual Compression of the Uterus for the Management of PPH (पी0पी0एच0 के प्रबंधन हेतु बच्चेदानी के बाएमेन्युल कम्प्रेशन मे सहायता करना/देखना)	1
42	Care of Mother with HIV (एच0आई0वी ग्रस्त माता की देखभाल)	1
43	Digital Removal of Retained Products of Conception for Incomplete Abortion (अपूर्ण गर्भपात के बचे हुए उत्पाद को डिजिटल तरीके से निकालना)	1
44	Provide Postabortion Care (गर्भपात के बाद देखभाल करना)	1
45	Counselling of Mother/Couples on Family Planning (माताओं/जोडो को परिवार नियोजन पर काउन्सिलिंग)	1
46	Prepare and Assist for Sterilisation (बंध्यीकरण के लिए तैयार एवं सहायता करना)	7
47	Prescription of Contraception (गर्भनिरोधन पर परामर्श)	1
48	Perform IUCD Insertions (आई0यू0 सी0डी0 लगाना)	2
49	Distribute Oral Pills (मौखिक गोलियों का वितरण)	5
50	Demonstrate the use of Condoms and distribute Condoms (कंडोम का प्रयोग सिखाना तथा वितरण)	5
51	Visual Inspection of the Cervix and Taking a Pap Smear Test (सर्विक्स का दृष्टिक निरीक्षण तथा पैप स्मियर जाँच लेना)	2
D.2	**IDENTIFY HIGH-RISK MOTHERS AND GIVE CARE IN COMMUNITY** (समुदाय में अधिक जोखिम वर्ग वाली माताओं को पहचानना तथा देखभाल करना)	
52	Case Study of Complicated Childbirth (जटिल शिशुजन्म पर केस अध्ययन)	1
53	Conduct a Village Meeting for Emergency Transport of Women at Risk (जोखिम वाली महिलाओं के आपातकालीन परिवहन हेतु एक ग्रामीण मीटिंग का संचालन)	1
54	Identify and Refer Women with Unwanted Pregnancy for MTP (एम0टी0पी0 के लिए अनचाहे गर्भ वाली महिला को पहचानना तथा रेफर करना)	1
55	Interview Women for Unsafe Motherhood and Abortion, and Mention Reasons (असुरक्षित मातृत्व और गर्भपात के लिए महिलाओ को साक्षात्कार और कारणों का उल्लेख)	10
56	Identify High-risk Mothers and Refer them to the Higher Center (अधिक जोखिम वाली माताओं को पहचानना तथा उन्हें उच्च केन्द्र पर संदर्भित करना)	5
57	Identify High-risk Newborns and Refer them to the Higher Center (अधिक जोखिम वाले नवजातों को पहचानना तथा उन्हें उच्च केन्द्र पर रेफर करना)	5

S. No	Competencies (कार्यनिर्वाह क्षमताएँ)	Number of Requirement
58	Counsel Eligible Couples on Different Methods of Contraception (गर्भनिरोधन के विभिन्न तरीकों पर योग्य जोडो को काउन्सिलिंग)	2
59	Perform IUCD Insertions (आई0यू0सी0डी0 लगाना)	2
60	Distribute Oral Pills (मौखिक गोलियों का वितरण)	5
61	Demonstrate the use of Condoms and Distribute Condoms (कंडोम का प्रयोग सिखाना तथा वितरण)	5
62	Visual Inspection of the Cervix and Taking a Pap Smear Test (सर्विक्स का दृष्टिक निरीक्षण तथा पैप स्मियर जाँच लेना)	2
VI	**HEALTH CENTER MANAGEMENT** (स्वास्थ्य केन्द्र प्रबन्धन)	
1	Organise a Set-up of Sub Center (उपकेन्द्र के सेटअप का आयोजन)	1
2	Maintain Vital Statistics Registers (जैविक आंकडो का रजिस्टर बनाना)	Each 1
3	Maintain Family Folders and Eligible Couple Register (परिवार फोल्डरों तथा योग्य जोड़ों के लिए रजिस्टर बनाना)	Each 1
4	Calculate and Maintain Indent and Stock Register (इंडेण्ट एवं स्टॉक रजिस्टर की गणना करना तथा बनाए रखना)	Each 1
5	Preparation of Reports (रिपोर्ट तैयार करना)	3
6	Screening Test (स्क्रीनिंग टेस्ट)	3
7	Referral Service (संदर्भित सेवा)	2
8	Organise and Participate in Various Clinic (विभिन्न चिकित्सालयों में सुनियोजन एवं भागीदारी)	3
9	Integrate/Participate in AYUSH Activity (आयुष के एकीकृत/गतिविधि मे भाग)	1
10	Conduct Health Camps (स्वास्थ्य शिविरो का आयोजन)	1
11	Peer Group Teaching (पीयर समूह को शिक्षण)	2
12	Display Health Messages at Sub Center (उपकेन्द्र पर स्वास्थ्य संदेशो का प्रदर्शन)	1
13	Observational Visit (ओबजर्वेशनल विज़िट)	3
14	Organise and Participate in all National Health Programme at Community/HSC/PHC/CHC (सामुदायिक राष्ट्रीय स्वास्थ्य कार्यक्रमो का आयोजन एवं भाग लेना/एच एस सी/पी एच सी/सी एच सी)	11

S. No	Competencies (कार्यनिर्वाह क्षमताएँ)	Number of Requirement
	INTERNSHIP (प्रशिक्षण)	
1	Examination of Antenatal Mother (एंटीनेटल माता का परीक्षण)	15
2	Pelvic Assessment and PV Examination (पेल्विक आंकलन एवं पी0वी0 परीक्षण)	5
3	Conducting Safe Deliveries (सुरक्षित प्रसव करवाना)	10
4	Assist in the Suturing of Episiotomies and Tears (एपीजियोट्मी एवं टीयर के टॉकें लगाने मे सहायता)	5
5	Provide Essential Care of Newborn (नवजात की अनिवार्य देखभाल प्रदान करना)	10
6	Basic Resuscitation of the Newborn (नवजात का बेसिक रिससीटेशन)	5
7	Care of Postnatal Mothers (प्रसव के बाद माताओं की देखभाल)	10
8	Care of Women with Abortion (गर्भपात वाली महिलाओ की देखभाल)	2
9	Prepare and Assist for Sterilisation (बंध्यीकरण के लिए तैयार एवं सहायता करना)	7
10	Perform IUCD Insertions (आई0यू0सी0डी0 लगाना)	3
11	Distribute Oral Pills (मौखिक गोलियों का वितरण)	5
12	Demonstrate the use of Condoms and Distribute it (कंडोम का प्रयोग सिखाना तथा वितरण)	5
13	Assessment and Care of Sick Neonates (as per the IMNCI Protocol) बीमार नवजातों का आंकलन तथा देखभाल (आई0एम0एन0सी0आई0 नियमों के अनुसार)	5
14	Assessment and Care of Sick Children (as per the IMNCI Protocol) बीमार बच्चों का आंकलन तथा देखभाल (आई0एम0एन0सी0आई0 नियमों के अनुसार)	5

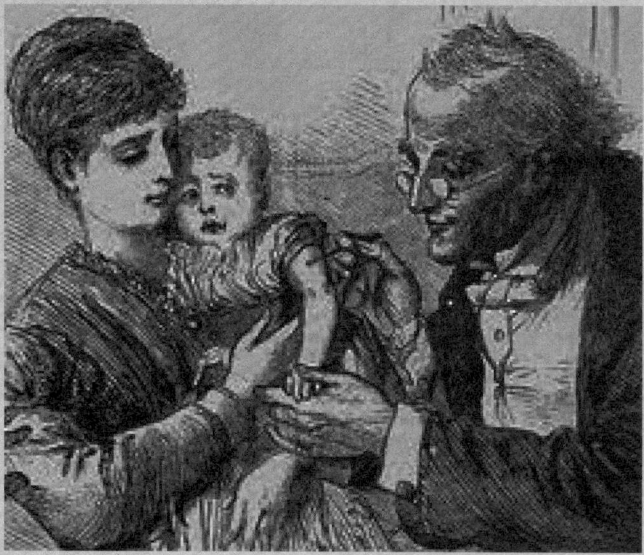

Competency Based Logbook for ANM

(कम्पीटेन्सी बेस्ड लॉगबुक फॉर एएनएम)

Section 1

Community Health Nursing
(सामुदायिक स्वास्थ्य परिचर्या)

CHAPTER 1

PLACEMENT: I YEAR **PRACTICAL: 110 (10 + 100) HOURS**

S. No	Competencies	Date of Demo	Sign of Nursing Tutor	Date of Return Demo	Sign of Clinical Supervisor
1	Survey (सर्वेक्षण)				
1.1	Community (समुदाय)				
1.2	Family Planning (परिवार नियोजन)				
1.3	Morbidity (रूग्णता)				
2	Mapping (मानचित्र बनाना)				
2.1	Village (गाँव)				
2.2	Slum (झुग्गी–झोंपड़ी)				
2.3	Resource (संसाधन)				
3	Prepare Health Organisation Chart (स्वास्थ्य संगठन चार्ट बनाना)				
3.1	Primary Health Center (प्राथमिक स्वास्थ्य केन्द्र)				
3.2	Community Health Center (सामुदायिक स्वास्थ्य केन्द्र)				
4	Home Visit (Family Health Assessment) होम विज़िट (पारिवारिक स्वास्थ्य का आंकलन)				
4.1					
4.2					
4.3					

S. No	Competencies	Date of Demo	Sign of Nursing Tutor	Date of Return Demo	Sign of Clinical Supervisor
4.4					
4.5					
5	Community Need Assessment (सामुदायिक आवश्यकताओं का आंकलन)				
6	Bag Technique (बैग तकनीक)				
6.1	Health Assessment (स्वास्थ्य का आंकलन)				
6.2	Nutritional Assessment (पोषण का आंकलन)				
6.3	Vital Signs and Blood Pressure (जैविक चिन्ह एवं रक्त दाब)				
6.4	Dressing (ड्रेसिंग)				
6.5	Administration of Medication (दवाईयो का एडमिनिस्ट्रेशन)				
(i)	Oral (मौखिक)				
(ii)	Intramuscular Injections (मांस पेशियों मे इंजेक्शन देना)				
(iii)	Intravenous Injections (नस मे इंजेक्शन लगाना)				
6.6	Steam Inhalation (भाप को लेना)				
6.7	Baby Bath (शिशु स्नान)				
6.8	Eye Care (आँखो की देखभाल)				
6.9	Cord Care (नाभी की देखभाल)				
6.10	Urine Test (मूत्र जाँच)				
(i)	Sugar (शुगर)				
(ii)	Albumin (एल्ब्यूमिन)				
7	Oral Rehydration Therapy (ORT) (मौखिक पुनर्जलीकरण थेरेपी)				

S. No	Competencies	Date of Demo	Sign of Nursing Tutor	Date of Return Demo	Sign of Clinical Supervisor
8	Assess Personal Hygiene of School Children (स्कूली बच्चों की व्यक्तिगत स्वच्छता का आंकलन)				
8.1					
8.2					
8.3					
8.4					
8.5					
9	Preparation of IEC Material (आई0ई0सी0 सामग्री की तैयारी)				
9.1	Chart (चार्ट)				
(i)	Panchayat Structure (पंचायत का ढाँचा)				
(ii)	Urban Ward (शहरी वार्ड)				
9.2	Flannel Graph (फ्लैनल ग्राफ)				
9.3	Flash Card (फ्लैश कार्ड)				
9.4	Flip Chart (फ्लिप चार्ट)				
9.5	Pamphlet (पर्चा)				
9.6	Poster (पोस्टर)				
9.7	Puppet Show (कठपुतली नाटृय)				
10	Conduct BCC Session (Role Play/folk Method) बी0सी0सी0 सत्र का संचालन (रोल प्ले / फोल्क मेथड)				
11	Prepare Health Education Plan (स्वास्थ्य शिक्षा योजना बनाना)				
12	Health Education (स्वास्थ्य शिक्षा)				
12.1	Individual (व्यक्तिगत)				
12.2	Group (समूह)				

S. No	Competencies	Date of Demo	Sign of Nursing Tutor	Date of Return Demo	Sign of Clinical Supervisor
12.3	Mass (बड़ा समूह)				
13	Counselling (समाधान)				
13.1	Preparation of Questionnaire (प्रश्नावली की तैयारी)				
13.2	Provide Counselling (काउन्सिलिंग देना)				
14	Participate in Health and Family Welfare Programme (स्वास्थ्य एवं परिवार कल्याण कार्यक्रम मे भाग लेना)				
15	Field Visit (ग्रामीण क्षैत्र का दौरा)				
15.1	Anganwadi (आँगनवाड़ी)				
15.2	Block Development Office (ब्लॉक डेवलपमेन्ट ऑफिस)				
15.3	Sub Center (उपकेन्द्र)				
15.4	Primary Health Center (प्राथमिक स्वास्थ्य केन्द्र)				
15.5	Community Health Center (सामुदायिक स्वास्थ्य केन्द्र)				
15.6	Red Cross Society (रेड क्रॉस सोसाइटी)				
15.7	Non-Governmental Organisation (गैर सरकारी संगठन)				
16	Group Work (सामूहिक कार्य)				
16.1	Nutrition Exhibition in School/Health Center (स्कूल/स्वास्थ्य केन्द्र में पोषण प्रदर्शनी)				
16.2	Cooking Demonstration (खाना पकाकर दिखाना)				
16.3	Prepare and Maintain a Nutrition Practical Book (न्यूट्रीशन की प्रैक्टिकल बुक बनाना)				

Signature of the Tutor/Class Coordinator **Signature of the Principal**

CHAPTER 2

Health Promotion
(स्वास्थ्य वर्धन)

PLACEMENT: I YEAR **PRACTICAL: 200 (20 + 180) HOURS**

S. NO	Competencies	Date of Demo	Sign of Nursing Tutor	Date of Return Demo	Sign of Clinical Supervisor
A	**NUTRITION** (पोषण)				
1	Nutritional Assessment (पोषण का आंकलन)				
1.1	Individual (Women/Child) (व्यक्तिगत महिलायें एवं बच्चे)				
1.2	Family (परिवार)				
2	Diet Planning (भोजन की योजना)				
2.1	Individual (Women/Child) व्यक्तिगत (महिलाऐं एवं बच्चे)				
2.2	Family (परिवार)				
3	Cooking Special Diet (विशेष भोजन पकाना)				
4	Nutrition Education to a Group (एक समूह को पोषण शिक्षा)				
5	Counselling on Nutrition (पोषण पर काउन्सिलिंग)				
5.1	Individual (व्यक्तिगत)				
5.2	Family (परिवार)				
5.3	Special Needs (विशेष आवश्यकताएँ)				
6	Exhibition on Balanced Diet (Using Raw Food Items) संतुलित आहार पर प्रदर्शनी (कच्चे खाद्य पदार्थो का प्रयोग)				

S. NO	Competencies	Date of Demo	Sign of Nursing Tutor	Date of Return Demo	Sign of Clinical Supervisor
7	Observational Visit (ओबसर्वेशनल विजिट)				
7.1	ICDS Project (आई0सी0डी0एस0 प्रोजेक्ट)				
7.2	Milk Pasteurization Plant (दुग्ध पॉस्च्युरीकरण प्लांट)				
B	**HUMAN BODY & HYGIENE** (मानव शरीर एवं साफ सफाई)				
8	Preparation of Anatomy Practical Book (एनाटमी की प्रैक्टिकल बुक बनाना)				
9	Care of Various Parts of Sick (रोगी के विभिन्न अंगो की देखभाल)				
9.1	Care of Skin (त्वचा की देखभाल)				
(i)	Bathing (स्नान)				
(ii)	Sponging (स्पन्जिंग)				
(iii)	Back Care (पीठ की देखभाल)				
(iv)	Care of Pressure Points (दाब बिंदुओ की देखभाल)				
(v)	Position Changing (पोजिशन बदलना)				
9.2	Care of Hair (बालों की देखभाल)				
(i)	Hair Wash (बाल धोना)				
(ii)	Hair Combing (बालों को कंघी करना)				
9.3	Care of Hands and Nails (हाथ एवं नाखुनों की देखभाल)				
(i)	Handwashing (हाथ धोना)				
(ii)	Nail Care (नाखुनों की देखभाल)				
9.4	Care of Eyes (Eye Wash) (आँखो की देखभाल)				
9.5	Care of Mouth (मुँह की देखभाल)				
10	Health Education on Menstrual Hygiene (मासिक चक्र के समय स्वच्छता पर स्वास्थ्य शिक्षा)				

S. NO	Competencies	Date of Demo	Sign of Nursing Tutor	Date of Return Demo	Sign of Clinical Supervisor
11	Counselling the Adolescence on Physiological Changes, Fulfillment of Basic Needs, Body Hygiene, and Healthy Life Styles (किशोरों को शारीरिक बदलाव, मूल आवश्यकताओं की भरपाई, शारीरिक स्वच्छता, एवं स्वास्थ्यप्रद जीवनशैली पर काउन्सिलिंग)				
C	**ENVIRONMENTAL SANITATION** (वातावरण की शुद्धता)				
12	Village Mapping (Water Source, Drains, Ponds and Contaminated Areas) गाँव का मानचित्र (जल स्रोत, नालियाँ तालाब एवं गन्दे क्षेत्र)				
13	Demonstrate Purification of Water (जल का शुद्धीकरण सिखाना)				
13.1	Home (Water Tank/Container) (घरेलू) (जल, टैंक/कंटेनर)				
13.2	Community (Well/ Tube Well) (सामुदायिक कुआँ/ट्यूबवेल)				
14	Guide or Plan Construction on Small Scale Soak Pit at School or Health Center (स्कूल या स्वास्थ्य केन्द्र पर छोटे स्केल का सोकपिट बनाने पर मार्गदर्शन या योजना बनाना)				
15	Health Education on use of Sanitary Latrine (सैनेट्री लैट्रिन के प्रयोग हेतु स्वास्थ्य शिक्षा)				
16	Field Visit (फील्ड विजिट)				
16.1	Water Purification Plant (जल शुद्धीकरण प्लांट)				
16.2	Sewage Treatment Plant and Sanitary Latrine (सीवेज ट्रीटमेन्ट प्लांट तथा सैनेट्री लैट्रीन)				
D	**MENTAL HEALTH** (मानसिक स्वास्थ्य)				
17	Assessment of Mental Health Status of an Individual (व्यक्ति के मानसिक स्वास्थ्य स्तर का आंकलन)				
17.1					
17.2					
18	Care of Mentally Challenged Patient (मानसिक रोगी की देखभाल)				
19	Counselling of Maladjusted Individual in Community (समुदाय मे मालएडजेस्टेड व्यक्ति की काउन्सिलिंग)				

S. NO	Competencies	Date of Demo	Sign of Nursing Tutor	Date of Return Demo	Sign of Clinical Supervisor
20	Care Plan for an Elderly Person at Home (एक वृद्ध व्यक्ति की घर पर देखभाल की योजना)				
21	Observational Visit (ओबजर्वेशनल विजिट)				
21.1	Mental Hospital (मानसिक अस्पताल)				
21.2	Old Age Home (वृद्ध लोगो का रैनबसेरा)				

Signature of the Tutor/Class Coordinator **Signature of the Principal**

PRACTICAL EXAMINATION	INTERNAL EXAMINER	EXTERNAL EXAMINER
Fist Appearance Signature: Date:		
Supplementary-1 Signature: Date:		
Supplementary-2 Signature: Date:		

CHAPTER 3

Primary Health Care Nursing-I
(प्राथमिक स्वास्थ्य देखभाल परिचर्या-I)

PLACEMENT: I YEAR **PRACTICAL: 390 (90 + 300) HOURS**

S. No	Competencies	Date of Demo	Sign of Nursing Tutor	Date of Return Demo	Sign of Clinical Supervisor
A	**INFECTION AND IMMUNIZATION** (संक्रमण एवं टीकाकरण)				
1	Sterilisation of Syringes and Needles (Using Pressure Cooker/Small Autoclave) सिरिंज एवं सुईयों का विसंक्रमण (प्रेशर कुकर/छोटे ओटोक्लेव के प्रयोग से)				
2	Vaccination Technique (टीकाकरण तकनीक)				
3	Assisting or Participating in Cold Chain System (शीतश्रृंखला प्रणाली में भागीदारी या सहायता)				
3.1	Maintenance of ILR (आई0एल0आर0 का रखरखाव)				
3.2	Preparation and Maintenance of ICE Pack/box (आईस पैक/बॉक्स बनाना एवं रखरखाव)				
3.3	Storage of Vaccines (टीकों का भण्डारण)				
3.4	Segregation of Unused Vaccines and its Containers (अप्रयुक्त टीके और उनके कंटेनर को अलग रखना)				
3.5	Calculation of Vaccine Requirement and Indenting (वैक्सीन की आवश्यकता की गणना एवं मांगपत्र)				
4	Participating in Immunization Camp (टीकाकरण कैम्प मे भाग लेना)				
5	Maintenance of Immunization Record (टीकाकरण रिकार्ड का रखरखाव)				
6	Preparation of Posture or Chart on Immunization Schedule (टीकाकरण सारिणी पर पोस्टर या चार्ट बनाना)				
7	Preparation of Malarial Slides (मलेरियल स्लाईडस् बनाना)				

S. No	Competencies	Date of Demo	Sign of Nursing Tutor	Date of Return Demo	Sign of Clinical Supervisor
8	Collection of Specimen (स्पेसीमेन इक्ठ्ठा करना)				
8.1	Blood (खून)				
8.2	Sputum (बलगम)				
8.3	Urine (मूत्र)				
8.4	Stool (मल)				
9	Biomedical Waste Management (जैव चिकित्सा अपशिष्ट का प्रबंधन)				
B	**COMMUNICABLE DISEASE** (संक्रमण रोग)				
10	Calculation of Morbidity and Mortality Rate (रूग्णता एवं मृत्यु दर की गणना)				
11	Preparation of Surveillance Report (सर्वेलेन्स रिपोर्ट बनाना)				
12	Standard Safety Measures in Nursing Practice (नर्सिंग प्रैक्टिस में स्टैन्डर्ड सेफ्टी मेज़र्स)				
13	Prepare Chart on Standard Safety Measures (स्टैन्डर्ड सेफ्टी मेज़र्स का चार्ट बनाना)				
14	Care of Communicable Disease (Child/Adult) (संक्रामक रोग की देखभाल बच्चे/वयस्क)				
14.1	Individual (व्यक्तिगत)				
14.2	Family (परिवार)				
15	Participate in Control of Epidemic and its Relief Work in the Community (समुदाय द्वारा महामारी के बचाव कार्य तथा नियंत्रण में भाग लेना)				
16	Conduct Health Education on Communicable Disease (संक्रामक रोग पर स्वास्थ्य शिक्षा का संचालन)				
17	Observational Visit (ओबजर्वेशनल विज़िट)				
17.1	Isolation Unit (आईसोलेशन युनिट)				
17.2	Infectious Disease Hospital/Center (संक्रामक रोग अस्पताल/केन्द्र)				

S. No	Competencies	Date of Demo	Sign of Nursing Tutor	Date of Return Demo	Sign of Clinical Supervisor
C	**COMMUNITY HEALTH PROBLEMS** (सामुदायिक स्वास्थ्य समस्याएँ)				
18	Vital Signs and BP (जैविक चिन्ह एवं बी0पी0)				
19	Urine Testing (मूत्र जाँच)				
19.1	Sugar (शुगर)				
19.2	Albumin (एल्ब्यूमिन)				
20	Steam Inhalation (स्टीम इन्हेलेशन)				
21	Oxygen Inhalation (ऑक्सीजन इन्हेलेशन)				
22	Instillation of Nasal Drops (नेजल ड्राप्स् डालना)				
23	Instillation of Eye Drop (नेत्र ड्राप्स् डालना)				
24	Local Hot Application (लोकल हॉट एप्लीकेशन)				
25	Local Cold Application (लोकल कोल्ड एप्लीकेशन)				
26	Urinary Catheterisation (यूरीनरी केथेटेराइजेशन)				
27	Plain Water Enema (प्लेन वॉटर एनीमा)				
28	Case Study on Patient With (रोगीयो पर केस अध्ययन)				
28.1					
28.2					
28.3					
28.4	Musculoskeletal Disease (मांसपेशियों, हड्डियों की बीमारी)				
28.5	Physically Challenged (शारीरिक रूप से विकलांग)				
D	**PRIMARY MEDICAL CARE** (प्राथमिक चिकित्सा से देखभाल)				
29	Calculation of Drug Dose and Conversion (ड्रग डोज़ का अनुमान एवं परिवर्तन करना)				

S. No	Competencies	Date of Demo	Sign of Nursing Tutor	Date of Return Demo	Sign of Clinical Supervisor
30	Preparation of List of Common Drug used in Sub Centre (Dosage, Route and Action, Indication, Contraindication, Side-Effect) उपकेन्द्र में उपयोग होने वाली दवाईयों की सूची बनाना (दवा की मात्रा, कहाँ से देना, प्रभाव)				
31	Administration of Medicine (दवाईयों का एडमिनिस्ट्रेशन)				
31.1	Local (लोकल)				
31.2	Oral (मौखिक)				
31.3	Subcutaneous (सबक्यूटेनियस)				
31.4	Intradermal (इंट्राडर्मल)				
31.5	Intramuscular (इंट्रामसक्यूलर)				
31.6	Intravenous (इंट्रावेनस)				
31.7	Rectal (रेक्टल)				
32	Preparation and Administration of IV Fluids (आई0वी0 द्रव की तैयारी करना एवं देना)				
32.1					
32.2					
32.3					
33	Preparation of Blood Transfusion as per the Protocol (नियमों के अनुसार रक्त चढाने की तैयारी)				
34	Drug Study on (दवाइयों का अध्ययन)				
34.1	Oral Drugs (मौखिक दवाईयां)				
34.2	Parenteral Drugs (पेरेनट्रल दवाईयां)				
34.3	Emergency Drugs (आपातकालीन दवाईयां)				
35	Participate in AYUSH Activity (आयुष कार्यवाही मे भाग लेना)				

S. No	Competencies	Date of Demo	Sign of Nursing Tutor	Date of Return Demo	Sign of Clinical Supervisor
E	**FIRST AID & REFERRAL** (प्राथमिक सहायता एवं संदर्भण)				
36	Care of Wound (घाव की देखभाल)				
37	Application of (लगाने की विधि)				
37.1	Nasal Pack (नेजल पैक)				
37.2	Tourniquet (टोर्नीकेट)				
37.3	Bandages (पट्टीयां)				
37.4	Splint (स्प्लिंट)				
37.5	Sling (स्लिंग)				
38	Insertion of Nasogastric Tube and Stomach Wash (नेसोगैसट्रिक ट्यूब डालना तथा स्टमक वॉश)				
39	Emergency Care (आपातकालीन देखभाल)				
39.1					
39.2					
39.3					
40	Basic Life Support (BLS) (बेसिक लाईफ सपोर्ट बी0एल0एस0)				
41	Transportation of Casualties (मरीजों का परिवहन)				

Signature of the Tutor/Class Coordinator **Signature of the Principal**

PRACTICAL EXAMINATION	INTERNAL EXAMINER	EXTERNAL EXAMINER
Fist Appearance Signature: Date:		
Supplementary-1 Signature: Date:		
Supplementary-2 Signature: Date:		

CHAPTER 4

Child Health Nursing
(शिशु स्वास्थ्य परिचर्या)

PLACEMENT: I YEAR **PRACTICAL: 180 (80 + 100) HOURS**

S. No	Competencies	Date of Demo	Sign of Nursing Tutor	Date of Return Demo	Sign of Clinical Supervisor
A	**CHILD HEALTH NURSING (HOSPITAL)** शिशु स्वास्थ्य परिचर्या (अस्पताल)				
1	Assess the Growth and Development of Children and Record on Chart (बच्चों की वृद्धि एवं विकास का आंकलन तथा चार्ट पर रिकार्ड)				
1.1	Infant (शिशु)				
(i)					
(ii)					
(iii)					
1.2	Under Five Children (पाँच वर्ष से कम आयु के बच्चे)				
(i)					
(ii)					
(iii)					
1.3	School Going Children (स्कूली बच्चें)				
(i)					
(ii)					
1.4	Adolescent (किशोर)				

S. No	Competencies	Date of Demo	Sign of Nursing Tutor	Date of Return Demo	Sign of Clinical Supervisor
(i)					
(ii)					
2	Assess the Health Status of Sick Children (बीमार बच्चों के स्वास्थ्य स्तर पर आंकलन)				
2.1	Fever (बुखार)				
(i)	Mercury Thermometer (मरकरी थर्मोमीटर)				
(ii)	Digital Thermometer (डिजिटल थर्मोमीटर)				
2.2	Hypothermia (Using Radiant Warmer) हाईपोथर्मिया (रेडियेंट वार्मर के प्रयोग से)				
2.3	Respiratory Difficulty (सांस मे कठिनाई)				
(i)	Respiratory Rate (श्वसन दर)				
(ii)	Patency of Airway (श्वसन नली का खुला होना)				
(iii)	Oxygen Saturation (Using Pulse Oximeter) आक्सीजन सैचुरेशन (पल्स् आक्सीमीटर के प्रयोग से)				
2.4	Respiratory Tract Infection (श्वसन तंत्र संक्रमण)				
2.5	Diarrhoea (अतिसार)				
2.6	Anemia (खून की कमी)				
2.7	Blood Glucose Level (रक्त ग्लूकोस स्तर)				
2.8	Jaundice (पीलिया)				
2.9	Feeding Problem (खाना खिलाने की समस्या)				
2.10	Malnutrition or Vitamin Deficiency (कुपोषण या विटामिन की कमी)				
3	Care of Common Childhood Illness (as per the IMNCI Protocol) बचपन के सामान्य रोगों की देखभाल (आई0एम0एन0सी0आई0 नियमों के अनुसार)				

S. No	Competencies	Date of Demo	Sign of Nursing Tutor	Date of Return Demo	Sign of Clinical Supervisor
3.1	Care of Fever (बुखार की देखभाल)				
3.2	Care of Hypothermia (हाईपोथर्मिया की देखभाल)				
3.3	Care of Respiratory Tract Infection (श्वसन तंत्र संक्रमण की देखभाल)				
3.4	Care of Respiratory Difficulty (श्वास की कठिनाई में देखभाल)				
(i)	Maintaining Patent Air Way by Using Electrical Suction Machine (इलैक्ट्रीकल सक्शन मशीन के प्रयोग द्वारा श्वसन नली को खुला करना)				
(ii)	Oxygen Therapy (आक्सीजन थेरेपी)				
(iii)	Nebulisation (नेब्युलाईजेशन)				
3.5	Care of Feeding Problem by (खिलाने की समस्या मे देखभाल)				
(i)	Insertion of Nasogastric Tube (नेसोगैस्ट्रिक टयूब डालना)				
(ii)	Nasogastric Tube Feeding (नेसोगैस्ट्रिक टयूब द्वारा खिलाना)				
3.6	Care of Diarrhoea (अतिसार की देखभाल)				
(i)	Administration of ORS (ओ0आर0एस0 देना)				
(ii)	Administration of Zinc Tablet (जिंक की गोली देना)				
(iii)	Administration of Antidiarrhoeal Drugs (एंटीडायरियल दवाई देना)				
3.7	Care of Jaundice by using Phototherapy Machine (फोटोथेरेपी मशीन के प्रयोग से पीलिया का इलाज)				
3.8	Care of Malnutrition or Vitamin Deficiency (कुपोषण या विटामिन की कमी में देखभाल)				
3.9	Care of Dysentry (पेचिश में देखभाल)				
3.10	Care of Convulsion (दौरे पड़ने में देखभाल)				
4	Infection Prevention Practice (संक्रमण रोकथाम प्रैक्टिस)				

S. No	Competencies	Date of Demo	Sign of Nursing Tutor	Date of Return Demo	Sign of Clinical Supervisor
4.1	Handwashing (हाथ धोना)				
4.2	Putting on and Removal of Gloves (दस्तानें पहनना एवं उतारना)				
4.3	Biomedical Segregation of Waste (जैव चिकित्सा कचरे का अलगाव)				
5	Care of Child Immunization (बच्चें के टीकाकरण की देखभाल)				
5.1	Care of BCG Vaccination (बी0सी0जी0 टीकाकरण में देखभाल)				
5.2	Care of OPV Vaccination (ओ0पी0वी0 टीकाकरण में देखभाल)				
5.3	Care of DPT Vaccination (डी0पी0टी0 टीकाकरण में देखभाल)				
5.4	Care of Hepatitis-B Vaccination (हेपाटाईटिस–बी0 टीकाकरण में देखभाल)				
5.5	Care of Measles Vaccination (मीसल्स् टीकाकरण में देखभाल)				
5.6	Care of TT Vaccination (टी0टी0 टीकाकरण में देखभाल)				
B	**CHILD HEALTH NURSING (COMMUNITY)** बाल स्वास्थ्य परिचर्या (सामुदायिक)				
6	Assess the Growth and Development of Children and Record on Chart (बच्चों की वृद्धि एवं विकास का आंकलन तथा चार्ट पर रिकार्ड)				
6.1	Infant (शिशु)				
(i)					
(ii)					
(iii)					
6.2	Under Five Children (पाँच वर्ष से कम आयु के बच्चे)				
(i)					
(ii)					
(iii)					

S. No	Competencies	Date of Demo	Sign of Nursing Tutor	Date of Return Demo	Sign of Clinical Supervisor
6.3	Schoolgoing Children (स्कूल जाने वाले बच्चे)				
(i)					
(ii)					
6.4	Adolescent (किशोर)				
(i)					
(ii)					
7	Assess the Health Status of Sick Children (बीमार बच्चों के स्वास्थ्य स्तर का आंकलन)				
7.1	Infant (शिशु)				
(i)					
(ii)					
(iii)					
7.2	Under Five Children (पाँच वर्ष से कम आयु के बच्चे)				
(i)					
(ii)					
(iii)					
7.3	Schoolgoing Children (स्कूली बच्चे)				
(i)					
(ii)					
7.4	Adolescent (किशोर)				
(i)					

S. No	Competencies	Date of Demo	Sign of Nursing Tutor	Date of Return Demo	Sign of Clinical Supervisor
(ii)					
8	Assess the Nutritional Status of the Children (बच्चों के पोषण स्तर का आंकलन)				
8.1	Protein Energy Malnutrition (प्रोटीन–उर्जा कुपोषण)				
8.2	Vitamin Deficiencies (विटामिन की कमी)				
9	Home Care of Common Childhood Illness (as per the IMNCI Protocol) बचपन मे होने वाले सामान्य रोगों की घर पर देखभाल (आई0एम0एन0सी0आई0 नियमों के अनुसार)				
9.1	Care of Cough (खॉसी में देखभाल)				
9.2	Care of Common Cold (जुखाम में देखभाल)				
9.3	Care of Fever (बुखार में देखभाल)				
9.4	Care of Diarrhoea (अतिसार में देखभाल)				
9.5	Care of Worm Infestation (कृमि संक्रमण में देखभाल)				
9.6	Care of Malnutrition (कुपोषण में देखभाल)				
9.7	Care of Vitamin Deficiency (विटामिन की कमी में देखभाल)				
9.8	Care for Allergy (एलर्जी में देखभाल)				
9.9	Care of Wound (घाव की देखभाल)				
9.10	Care of Malaria (मलेरिया में देखभाल)				
10	Identify and Refer the Children at Risk (रिस्क वाले बच्चों को पहचानना एवं रेफर करना)				
11	Infection Prevention Practice (संक्रमण निरोधक प्रैक्टिस)				
11.1	Handwashing (हाथ धोना)				
11.2	Preparation of 0.5% Chlorine Solution (0.5 क्लोरिन घोल बनाना)				

S. No	Competencies	Date of Demo	Sign of Nursing Tutor	Date of Return Demo	Sign of Clinical Supervisor
12	Health Education (स्वास्थ्य शिक्षा)				
12.1	Mothers (माताऐं)				
(i)	Exclusive Breastfeeding (अनन्य स्तनपान)				
(ii)	Breastfeeding Technique (स्तनपान तकनीक)				
(iii)	Preparation of ORS (ओ0आर0एस0 बनाना)				
(iv)	Preparation and Feeding of Complementary Feeds/Food (पूरक आहार बनाना एवं खिलाना)				
12.2	School Children (स्कूली बच्चे)				
(i)	Personal Hygiene (शारीरिक शिक्षा)				
(ii)	Road Safety (सड़क सुरक्षा)				
13	Prepare Poster (पोस्टर बनाना)				
13.1	Growth and Development (Birth to Adolescent) वृद्धि एवं विकास (जन्म से किशोरावस्था)				
13.2	Prevention on Common Accidents in Children (बच्चों की सामान्य दुर्घटनाओं से रोकथाम)				
13.3	Menstrual Cycle (मासिक चक्र)				
13.4	Physical Changes in Adolescence (किशोरावस्था मे शारिरिक बदलाव)				
14	Counselling (काउन्सिलिंग)				
14.1	Mothers (माताएँ)				
14.2	Children (बच्चें)				
14.3	Adolescent (किशोर)				
15	Survey on Child Labour in the Community (समुदाय में बाल मजदूरी पर सर्वेक्षण)				
16	Observational Visit to School (स्कूल पर ओबजर्वेशनल विजिट)				

S. No	Competencies	Date of Demo	Sign of Nursing Tutor	Date of Return Demo	Sign of Clinical Supervisor
17	Organise or Participate in School Health Service (स्कूल स्वास्थ्य सेवाओं मे भागेदारी या संगठन)				
18	Maintain School Health Record (स्कूल स्वास्थ्य रिकार्ड बनाना)				
18.1					
18.2					
18.3					
18.4					
18.5					
19	Case Studies (Hospital/ Community) केस स्टडीज़ (अस्पताल / समुदाय)				
19.1	Infant (शिशु)				
19.2	Under Five Children (पाँच वर्ष से कम आयु के बच्चे)				
19.3	Schoolgoing (स्कूली बच्चे)				
19.4	Adolescent (किशोर)				

Signature of the Tutor/Class Coordinator **Signature of the Principal**

PRACTICAL EXAMINATION	INTERNAL EXAMINER	EXTERNAL EXAMINER
Fist Appearance Signature: Date:		
Supplementary-1 Signature: Date:		
Supplementary-2 Signature: Date:		

Section 2

CHAPTER 5

Midwifery
(प्रसूति विद्या)

PLACEMENT: II YEAR **PRACTICAL: 380 (220 + 160) HOURS**

S. No	Competencies	Date of Demo	Sign of Nursing Tutor	Date of Return Demo	Sign of Clinical Supervisor
A.1	**CARE OF ANTENATAL MOTHERS IN HOSPITAL** (अस्पताल में गर्भवती महिला की देखभाल)				
1	Preconception Counselling (गर्भधारण से पूर्व कउन्सिलिंग)				
1.1					
1.2					
2	Detecting Pregnancy by Using Pregnancy Testing Kit (गर्भ जाँच किट के प्रयोग से गर्भ का पता लगाना)				
2.1					
2.2					
3	Calculation of EDD (ई0डी0डी0 अनुमान लगाना)				
3.1					
3.2					
4	Registration of Antenatal Mothers (प्रसव से पूर्व माताओं का पंजीकरण)				
4.1					
4.2					
5	Haemoglobin Estimation (हीमोग्लोबिन की जाँच)				

S. No	Competencies	Date of Demo	Sign of Nursing Tutor	Date of Return Demo	Sign of Clinical Supervisor
5.1					
5.2					
6	Urine Test (मूत्र जाँच)				
6.1	Sugar (शुगर)				
6.2	Albumin (एल्ब्यूमिन)				
7	Antenatal Examination (Name – Gravida/Condition) प्रसव पूर्व परिक्षण (नाम–ग्रैविडा / कंडीशन)				
7.1					
7.2					
7.3					
7.4					
7.5					
7.6					
7.7					
7.8					
7.9					
7.10					
7.11					
7.12					
7.13					

S. No	Competencies	Date of Demo	Sign of Nursing Tutor	Date of Return Demo	Sign of Clinical Supervisor
7.14					
7.15					
8	Supplementation of IFA (Iron & Folic Acid) आई0एफ0ए0 के पूरक (आयरन एवं फॉलिक एसिड)				
8.1					
8.2					
8.3					
8.4					
8.5					
8.6					
8.7					
8.8					
8.9					
8.10					
9	Administration of TT Injection (टी0टी0 इंजेक्शन लगाना)				
9.1					
9.2					
9.3					
9.4					
9.5					

S. No	Competencies	Date of Demo	Sign of Nursing Tutor	Date of Return Demo	Sign of Clinical Supervisor
9.6					
9.7					
9.8					
9.9					
9.10					
A.2	**CARE OF ANTENATAL MOTHERS IN COMMUNITY** (समुदाय में गर्भवती से पूर्व माताओं की देखभाल करना)				
10	Registration of Vital Events Registers (जैविक घटनाओं के रजिस्टर का पंजीकरण)				
11	Assist in Management of Vital Events Registers (जैविक घटनाओं के रजिस्टर के प्रबंधन में सहायता)				
12	Participate in Antenatal Clinics in the Sub Center (उपकेन्द्र पर एंटीनेटल क्लिनिक मे भाग लेना)				
13	Antenatal Examination (Name – Gravida/Condition) (प्रसवपूर्व परीक्षण) (नाम– ग्रैविडा/कंडीशन)				
13.1					
13.2					
13.3					
13.4					
13.5					
14	Malaria Testing for Pregnant Mothers (गर्भवती माताओं की मलेरिया जाँच)				
15	Counselling (काउन्सिलिंग)				
15.1	Birth Preparedness (जन्म की तैयारी)				
15.2	Complication Readiness (जटिलताओं के लिए तैयार रहना)				

S. No	Competencies	Date of Demo	Sign of Nursing Tutor	Date of Return Demo	Sign of Clinical Supervisor
15.3	Diet and Rest (भोजन एवं आराम)				
15.4	Infant Feeding (शिशु को खिलाना)				
15.5	Sex During Pregnancy (गर्भ के दौरान संभोग)				
15.6	Domestic Violence (घरेलू हिंसा)				
15.7	Contraception (गर्भ निरोधन)				
B	**INTRANATAL CARE IN HOSPITAL AND COMMUNITY** (अस्पताल में गर्भवती की देखभाल)				
16	Maintain Midwifery Case Book (मिडवाइफरी केस बुक बनाना)				
17	Assessment and Care of First Stage of Labour (PV Examination) प्रसव के पहले चरण का आंकलन एवं देखभाल (पी0वी0 परिक्षण)				
17.1					
17.2					
17.3					
17.4					
17.5					
18	Plotting the Partograph (पोर्टोग्राफ भरना)				
18.1					
18.2					
18.3					
18.4					
18.5					

S. No	Competencies	Date of Demo	Sign of Nursing Tutor	Date of Return Demo	Sign of Clinical Supervisor
19	Assessment and Care of Second and Third Stage of Labour – Conducting Safe Deliveries (प्रसव के दूसरे तथा तीसरे चरण का आंकलन तथा देखभाल सुरक्षित प्रसव करवाना)				
19.1					
19.2					
19.3					
19.4					
19.5					
19.6					
19.7					
19.8					
19.9					
19.10					
20	Assist in the Suturing (Episiotomies and Tears) टांके लगाने में सहायता (एपीजियोटमी एवं टीयर)				
20.1					
20.2					
20.3					
20.4					
20.5					
21	Assist in Management of Intranatal Complications (प्रसवोत्तर जटिलताओ के प्रबंधन मे सहायता)				

S. No	Competencies	Date of Demo	Sign of Nursing Tutor	Date of Return Demo	Sign of Clinical Supervisor
C.1	**CARE OF POSTNATAL MOTHERS IN HOSPITAL** (अस्पताल में प्रसव के बाद माताओं की देखभाल)				
22	Provide Essential Care of the Newborn (नवजात को अतिआवश्यक देखभाल प्रदान करना)				
22.1					
22.2					
22.3					
22.4					
22.5					
22.6					
22.7					
22.8					
22.9					
22.10					
23	Basic Resuscitation of the Newborn (नवजात का बेसिक रिससीटेशन)				
23.1					
23.2					
23.3					
23.4					
23.5					
24	Care of Postnatal Mothers (प्रसव के बाद माताओं की देखभाल)				
24.1					

S. No	Competencies	Date of Demo	Sign of Nursing Tutor	Date of Return Demo	Sign of Clinical Supervisor
24.2					
24.3					
24.4					
24.5					
24.6					
24.7					
24.8					
24.9					
24.10					
25	Health Education (स्वास्थ्य शिक्षा)				
25.1	Group (समूह)				
(i)					
(ii)					
(iii)					
25.2	Individual (व्यक्तिगत)				
(i)					
(ii)					
(iii)					
26	Counselling (काउन्सिलिंग)				

S. No	Competencies	Date of Demo	Sign of Nursing Tutor	Date of Return Demo	Sign of Clinical Supervisor
26.1	Breastfeeding (स्तनपान)				
26.2	Prevention and Management of Breastfeeding Problems (स्तनपान की परेशानीयो की रोकथाम एवं प्रबंधन)				
26.3	Kangaroo Care (कंगारू देखभाल)				
27	Follow Biomedical Waste Management (जैव कचरा प्रबंधन)				
27.1	Labour Room (प्रसूति कक्ष)				
27.2	Sub Center (उपकेन्द्र)				
C.2	**CARE OF POSTNATAL MOTHERS IN COMMUNITY** (समुदाय में प्रसव के बाद माताओं की देखभाल)				
28	Follow-up of Postnatal Mothers (प्रसव के बाद माताओं की देखभाल)				
28.1					
28.2					
28.3					
28.4					
28.5					
28.6					
28.7					
28.8					
28.9					
28.10					
29	Care of Newborn (नवजात की देखभाल)				
29.1					

S. No	Competencies	Date of Demo	Sign of Nursing Tutor	Date of Return Demo	Sign of Clinical Supervisor
29.2					
29.3					
29.4					
29.5					
29.6					
29.7					
29.8					
29.9					
29.10					
30	Conduct Health Education (स्वास्थ्य शिक्षा का संचालन)				
30.1	Individual (व्यक्ति)				
(i)					
(ii)					
30.2	Group (समूह)				
(i)					
(ii)					
D.1	**IDENTIFY HIGH-RISK MOTHERS AND GIVE CARE IN HOSPITAL** (अस्पताल में अधिक जोखिम वर्ग वाली माताओं को पहचानना तथा देखभाल करना)				
31	Identify High-risk Mothers and Give Care (अधिक जोखिम वर्ग वाली माताओं को पहचानना तथा देखभाल करना)				
31.1					

S. No	Competencies	Date of Demo	Sign of Nursing Tutor	Date of Return Demo	Sign of Clinical Supervisor
31.2					
32	Prepare for Caesarean Sections (सिज़ेरियन सेक्शन की तैयारी)				
32.1					
32.2					
33	Observe Caesarean Section (सिज़ेरियन सेक्शन देखना)				
33.1					
33.2					
34	Observe Abnormal Deliveries (असाधारण प्रसव देखना)				
34.1					
34.2					
34.3					
34.4					
34.5					
35	Prepare for MTP and Observe Procedure (एम0टी0पी0 की तैयारी तथा प्रोसीजर देखना)				
35.1					
35.2					
36	Care of Women with Abortion (गर्भपात वाली महिलाओं की देखभाल)				
36.1					
36.2					

S. No	Competencies	Date of Demo	Sign of Nursing Tutor	Date of Return Demo	Sign of Clinical Supervisor
37	Starting Intravenous Line (इंट्रावीनस लाईन शुरू करना)				
37.1					
37.2					
38	Urinary Catheterisation in Women (महिलाओं में युरीनरी कैथेट्रेराइजेशन)				
38.1					
38.2					
39	Preparation and Administration of Magnesium Sulphate Injection (मैग्निशियम सल्फेट इंजेक्शन तैयार करना तथा लगाना)				
40	Preparation and Administration of Oxytocin Drip (आक्सीटोसिन ड्रिप तैयार करना तथा देना)				
41	Assist/Observe Bimanual Compression of the Uterus for the Management of PPH (पी0पी0एच0 के प्रबंधन हेतु बच्चेदानी के बाएमेन्युल कम्प्रेशन मे सहायता करना/देखना)				
42	Care of Mother with HIV (एच0आई0वी0 ग्रस्त माता की देखभाल)				
43	Digital Removal of Retained Products of Conception for Incomplete Abortion (अपूर्ण गर्भपात के बचे हुए उत्पाद को डिजिटल तरीके से निकालना)				
44	Provide Postabortion Care (गर्भपात के बाद देखभाल करना)				
45	Counselling of Mother /Couples on Family Planning (माताओं/जोडो को परिवार नियोजन पर काउन्सिलिंग)				
46	Prepare and Assist for Sterilisation (बंध्यीकरण के लिए तैयार एवं सहायता करना)				
46.1	Female Case (महिला केस)				
(i)					

S. No	Competencies	Date of Demo	Sign of Nursing Tutor	Date of Return Demo	Sign of Clinical Supervisor
(ii)					
(iii)					
(iv)					
(v)					
46.2	Male Case (पुरूष केस)				
(vi)					
(vii)					
47	Prescription of Contraception (गर्भनिरोधन पर परामर्श)				
48	Perform IUCD Insertions (आई0यू0सी0डी0 लगाना)				
48.1					
48.2					
49	Distribute Oral Pills (मौखिक गोलियों का वितरण)				
49.1					
49.2					
49.3					
49.4					
49.5					
50	Demonstrate the use of Condoms and Distribute Condoms (कंडोम का प्रयोग सिखाना तथा वितरण)				
50.1					

S. No	Competencies	Date of Demo	Sign of Nursing Tutor	Date of Return Demo	Sign of Clinical Supervisor
50.2					
50.3					
50.4					
50.5					
51	Visual Inspection of the Cervix and Taking a Pap Smear Test (सर्विक्स का दृष्टिक निरीक्षण तथा पैप स्मियर जाँच लेना)				
51.1					
51.2					
D.2	**IDENTIFY HIGH-RISK MOTHERS AND GIVE CARE IN COMMUNITY** (समुदाय में अधिक जोखिम वर्ग वाली माताओं को पहचानना तथा देखभाल करना)				
52	Case Study of Complicated Childbirth (जटिल शिशुजन्म पर केस अध्ययन)				
53	Conduct a Village Meeting for Emergency Transport of Women at Risk (जोखिम वाली महिलाओं के आपातकालीन परिवहन हेतु एक ग्रामीण मीटिंग का संचालन)				
54	Identify and Refer Women with Unwanted Pregnancy for MTP (एम0टी0पी0 के लिए अनचाहे गर्भ वाली महिला को पहचानना तथा रेफर करना)				
55	Interview Women for Unsafe Motherhood and Abortion, and Mention Reasons (असुरक्षित मातृत्व और गर्भपात के लिए महिलाओं को साक्षात्कार और कारणों का उल्लेख)				
55.1					
55.2					
55.3					
55.4					

S. No	Competencies	Date of Demo	Sign of Nursing Tutor	Date of Return Demo	Sign of Clinical Supervisor
55.5					
55.6					
55.7					
55.8					
55.9					
55.10					
56	Identify High-risk Mothers and Refer them to the Higher Center (अधिक जोखिम वाली माताओं को पहचानना तथा उन्हें उच्च केन्द्र पर संदर्भित करना)				
56.1					
56.2					
56.3					
56.4					
56.5					
57	Identify High-risk Newborns and Refer them to the Higher Center (अधिक जोखिम वाले नवजातों को पहचानना तथा उन्हें उच्च केन्द्र पर रेफर करना)				
57.1					
57.2					
57.3					
57.4					

S. No	Competencies	Date of Demo	Sign of Nursing Tutor	Date of Return Demo	Sign of Clinical Supervisor
57.5					
58	Counsel Eligible Couples on Different Methods of Contraception (गर्भनिरोधन के विभिन्न तरीकों पर योग्य जोड़ो को काउन्सिलिंग)				
58.1					
58.2					
59	Perform IUCD Insertions आई0यू0सी0डी0 लगाना				
59.1					
59.2					
60	Distribute Oral Pills (मौखिक गोलियों का वितरण)				
60.1					
60.2					
60.3					
60.4					
60.5					
61	Demonstrate the use of Condoms and Distribute Condoms (कंडोम का प्रयोग सिखाना तथा वितरण)				
61.1					
61.2					
61.3					
61.4					

S. No	Competencies	Date of Demo	Sign of Nursing Tutor	Date of Return Demo	Sign of Clinical Supervisor
61.5					
62	Visual Inspection of the Cervix and Taking a Pap Smear Test (सर्विक्स का दृष्टिक निरीक्षण तथा पैप स्मियर जाँच लेना)				
62.1					
62.2					

Signature of the Tutor/Class Coordinator

Signature of the Principal

PRACTICAL EXAMINATION	INTERNAL EXAMINER	EXTERNAL EXAMINER
Fist Appearance Signature: Date:		
Supplementary-1 Signature: Date:		
Supplementary-2 Signature: Date:		

CHAPTER 6

Health Center Management
(स्वास्थ्य केन्द्र प्रबंधन)

PLACEMENT: II YEAR **PRACTICAL: 60 HOURS**

S. No	Competencies	Date of Demo	Sign of Nursing Tutor	Date of Return Demo	Sign of Clinical Supervisor
1	Organise a Set-up of Sub Center (उपकेन्द्र के सेटअप का आयोजन)				
2	Maintain Vital Statistics Registers (जैविक आंकडो का रजिस्टर बनाना)				
3	Maintain Family Folders and Eligible Couple Register (परिवार फोल्डरों तथा योग्य जोड़ों के लिए रजिस्टर बनाना)				
4	Calculate and Maintain Indent and Stock Register (इंडेण्ट एवं स्टॉक रजिस्टर की गणना करना तथा बनाए रखना)				
5	Preparation of Report (रिपोर्ट तैयार करना)				
5.1	Daily Report (दैनिक रिपोर्ट)				
5.2	Weekly Report (साप्ताहिक रिपोर्ट)				
5.3	Monthly Report (मासिक रिपोर्ट)				
6	Screening Test (स्क्रीनिंग टेस्ट)				
6.1	Tuberculosis (क्षयरोग)				
6.2	Malaria (मलेरिया)				
6.3	Leprosy (कुष्ठरोग)				
7	Referral Service (संदर्भित सेवा)				
7.1	Refer the Patient to District/ Regional Hospital (रोगी को जिला/क्षेत्रीय अस्पताल पर रेफर करना)				

S. No	Competencies	Date of Demo	Sign of Nursing Tutor	Date of Return Demo	Sign of Clinical Supervisor
7.2	Refer the Patient to PHC/CHC (रोगी को पी0एच0सी0 / सी0एच0सी0 पर रेफर करना)				
8	Organise and Participate in Various Clinic (विभिन्न चिकित्सालयों में सुनियोजन एवं भागीदारी)				
8.1					
8.2					
8.3					
9	Integrate/Participate in AYUSH Activity (आयुष के एकीकृत / गतिविधि मे भाग)				
10	Conduct Health Camps (स्वास्थ्य शिविरों का आयोजन)				
11	Peer Group Teaching on (पीयर समूह को शिक्षण)				
11.1	DOTS (डी0ओ0टी0एस0)				
11.2	MDT (एम0डी0टी0)				
12	Display Health Messages at Sub Center (उपकेन्द्र पर स्वास्थ्य संदेशो का प्रदर्शन)				
13	Observational Visit (ओबजर्वेशनल विज़िट)				
13.1	NGO (गैर सरकारी संगठन)				
13.2	Tuberculosis Clinic (DOTS programme) (क्षयरोग क्लिनिक) (डी0ओ0टी0एस0 कार्यक्रम)				
13.3	Leprosy Clinic (MDT) (कुष्ठरोग क्लिनिक) (एम0डी0टी0)				
14	Organise and Participate in All National Health Programme at Community/HSC/PHC/CHC (सामुदायिक राष्ट्रीय स्वास्थ्य कार्यक्रमो का आयोजन एवं भाग लेना / एच एस सी / पी एच सी / सी एच सी)				
14.1	World TB Day (विश्व टी0बी0 दिवस)				
14.2	World Blood Donation Day (विश्व रक्तदान दिवस)				
14.3	World Breastfeeding Week (विश्व स्तनपान सप्ताह)				

S. No	Competencies	Date of Demo	Sign of Nursing Tutor	Date of Return Demo	Sign of Clinical Supervisor
14.4	National Nutrition Week (राष्ट्रीय पोषण सप्ताह)				
14.5	World Mental Health Day (विश्व मानसिक स्वास्थ्य दिवस)				
14.6	World Polio Day (विश्व पोलियो दिवस)				
14.7	World Immunization Day (विश्व टीकाकरण दिवस)				
14.8	World Diabetes Day (विश्व मधुमेह दिवस)				
14.9	World AIDS Day (विश्व एडस् दिवस)				
14.10	National Prevention Population Day (राष्ट्रीय जनसंख्या रोकथाम दिवस)				
14.11	World Patient Safety Day (विश्व रोगी सुरक्षा दिवस)				

Signature of the Tutor/Class Coordinator

Signature of the Principal

PRACTICAL EXAMINATION	INTERNAL EXAMINER	EXTERNAL EXAMINER
Fist Appearance Signature: Date:		
Supplementary-1 Signature: Date:		
Supplementary-2 Signature: Date:		

Section 3

CHAPTER 7

Midwifery, Child Health Nursing, Community Health and Health Center Management
(प्रसूति विद्या, शिशु स्वास्थ्य परिचर्या, समुदाय स्वास्थ्य एवम् स्वास्थ्य केन्द्र प्रबंधन)

PLACEMENT: II YEAR (INTERNSHIP) **PRACTICAL: 880 (480 + 240 + 160) HOURS**

S. No	Competencies	Hospital or Community	Date of Return Demonstration	Sign of Clinical Supervisor
1	Examination of Antenatal Mother (एंटीनेटल माता का परीक्षण)			
1.1				
1.2				
1.3				
1.4				
1.5				
1.6				
1.7				
1.8				
1.9				
1.10				
1.11				
1.12				
1.13				
1.14				
1.15				

S. No	Competencies	Hospital or Community	Date of Return Demonstration	Sign of Clinical Supervisor
2	Pelvic Assessment & PV Examination (पेल्विक आंकलन एवं पी0वी0 परीक्षण)			
2.1				
2.2				
2.3				
2.4				
2.5				
3	Conducting Safe Deliveries (सुरक्षित प्रसव करवाना)			
3.1				
3.2				
3.3				
3.4				
3.5				
3.6				
3.7				
3.8				
3.9				
3.10				
4	Assist in the Suturing of Episiotomies and Tears (एपीजियोट्मी एवं टीयर के टॉकें लगाने मे सहायता)			
4.1				
4.2				
4.3				

S. No	Competencies	Hospital or Community	Date of Return Demonstration	Sign of Clinical Supervisor
4.4				
4.5				
5	Provide Essential Care of Newborn (नवजात की अनिवार्य देखभाल प्रदान करना)			
5.1				
5.2				
5.3				
5.4				
5.5				
5.6				
5.7				
5.8				
5.9				
5.10				
6	Basic Resuscitation of the Newborn (नवजात का बेसिक रिससीटेशन)			
6.1				
6.2				
6.3				
6.4				
6.5				
7	Care of Postnatal Mothers (प्रसव के बाद माताओं की देखभाल)			
7.1				
7.2				

S. No	Competencies	Hospital or Community	Date of Return Demonstration	Sign of Clinical Supervisor
7.3				
7.4				
7.5				
7.6				
7.7				
7.8				
7.9				
7.10				
8	Care of Women with Abortion (गर्भपात वाली महिलाओ की देखभाल)			
8.1				
8.2				
9	Prepare and Assist for Sterilisation (बंध्यीकरण के लिए तैयार एवं सहायता करना)			
9.1	Female Cases (महिला केस)			
(i)				
(ii)				
(iii)				
(iv)				
(v)				
9.2	Male Cases (पुरूष केस)			
(i)				
(ii)				

S. No	Competencies	Hospital or Community	Date of Return Demonstration	Sign of Clinical Supervisor
10	Perform IUCD Insertions (आई0यू0सी0डी0 लगाना)			
10.1				
10.2				
10.3				
11	Distribute Oral Pills (मौखिक गोलियो का वितरण)			
11.1				
11.2				
11.3				
11.4				
11.5				
12	Demonstrate the use of Condoms and Distribute it (कंडोम का प्रयोग सिखाना तथा वितरण)			
12.1				
12.2				
12.3				
12.4				
12.5				
13	Assessment and Care of Sick Neonates (as per the IMNCI Protocol) (बीमार नवजातों का आंकलन तथा देखभाल) (आई0एम0एन0सी0आई0 नियमों के अनुसार)			
13.1				
13.2				
13.3				

S. No	Competencies	Hospital or Community	Date of Return Demonstration	Sign of Clinical Supervisor
13.4				
13.5				
14	Assessment and Care of Sick Children (as per the IMNCI Protocol) (बीमार बच्चों का आंकलन तथा देखभाल) (आई0एम0एन0सी0आई0 नियमों के अनुसार)			
14.1				
14.2				
14.3				
14.4				
14.5				

Signature of the Tutor/Class Coordinator **Signature of the Principal**

FIRST YEAR CLINICAL EXPERIENCES

S. No	SUBJECTS	CLASS ROOM		HOSPITAL		COMMUNITY	
		Required (Hours)	Attended (Hours)	Required (Hours)	Attended (Hours)	Required (Hours)	Attended (Hours)
I	**Community Health Nursing**	**50**		**10**		**100**	
II	**Health Promotion**	**75**		**20**		**180**	
A	Nutrition	30					
B	Human Body and Hygiene	20					
C	Environmental Sanitation	15					
D	Mental Health	10					
III	**Primary Health Care Nursing-I**	**150**		**90**		**300**	
A	Infection and Immunization	20					
B	Communicable Disease	25					
C	Community Health Problems	50					
D	Primary Medical Care	20					
E	First Aid and Referral	35					
IV	**Child Health Nursing**	**110**		**80**		**100**	
Total Hours		**385**		**200**		**680**	

Signature of the Class Coordinator **Signature of the Principal**

SECOND YEAR CLINICAL EXPERIENCES

S. No	SUBJECTS	CLASS ROOM		HOSPITAL		COMMUNITY	
		Required (Hours)	Attended (Hours)	Required (Hours)	Attended (Hours)	Required (Hours)	Attended (Hours)
VI	Health Center Management	40				60	
	Total Hours	200		220		220	
	INTERNSHIP PERIOD						
I	**Midwifery**			240		240	
	Antenatal Ward			40			
	Intranatal/Lobour Room			120			
	Postnatal Ward			40			
	Neonatal Ward			40			
II	**Child Health Nursing**			80		160	
III	**Community Health and Health Center Management**					160	
	Total Hours			320		560	

Signature of the Class Coordinator **Signature of the Principal**

FIRST YEAR

Ms/Mrs ____ has been completed her first year clinical requirements with adequate knowledge and satisfactory skill.

PRINCIPAL

SECOND YEAR

Ms/Mrs. ____ has been completed her second year clinical requirements with adequate knowledge and satisfactory Skill.

PRINCIPAL

INTERNSHIP PERIOD

Ms/Mrs. ____ had been completed her internship period from ______________________ to ______________________, with adequate competencies in all Specialized health and family welfare activities.

PRINCIPAL